YOUR KNOWLEDGE HAS VALUE

Primary health care services delivery. Issues and challenges

A case of Benue State in North Central Nigeria

Makar Linus Iornenge

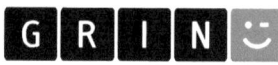

Bibliographic information published by the German National Library:

The German National Library lists this publication in the National Bibliography; detailed bibliographic data are available on the Internet at http://dnb.dnb.de.

ISBN: 9783346273505
This book is also available as an ebook.

PRIMARY HEALTH CARE SERVICES DELIVERY: ISSUES AND CHALLENGES:

A   CASE   OF   BENUE   STATE ,NORTH CENTRAL NIGERIA

BY

MAKAR LINUS IORNENGE,BSC,MPA,M.A,M.SC,(BSU)Ph.D IN VIEW(EBSU)

Abstract

Quality health is a fundamental right of all Nigerian citizens. While primary health care (PHC) centers are relatively uniformly distributed throughout local government areas (LGAs) in Nigeria, the rural people tend to underuse the basic health services. This paper examines primary health care delivery,issues and challenges in PHC and outlines strategies to enhance the utilization of health services by rural people in Benue State. The responsibility for perpetuating the existing low use of PHC services should be held by PHC policy makers and LGA. Responsible health personnel can build a new social order, based on greater equity and human dignity, in which health for all by the year 2015, including that of rural populations, will no more be a dream but a reality. Capacity building and empowerment of communities through orientation, mobilization and community organization as regards training, information sharing and continuous dialogue, could further enhance the utilization of PHC services by rural populations.

Table of Contents

SECTION ONE: INTRODUCTION

1.1 Background to the study

Improving health throughout the world is a gigantic task requiring global cooperation. The international health care system was first recognized at the first international scientific conference in 1851 (Shunom, 2006), after which the World Health Organization (WHO) introduced a system of cooperation against the spread of diseases. A WHO conference held in Alma-Ata in 1978, proclaimed Primary Health Care (PHC), as a concept that calls for the overall promotion of health by supporting the individual, the family and the community, by defining the active participation of the community, their needs and ways to meet them (Ogbole, 1981). Studies have shown that the problems confronting Nigeria in areas of health are many, ranging from poor finance, equipment, shortage of manpower to the unwillingness of few health professionals to work in rural areas (Brieger, 1980; Obionu, 2007). The health care delivery system which gives emphasis on erection of magnificent buildings and provision of sophisticated equipment to serve a few urban dwellers is known to be inadequate. Investing on such health delivery system will not ensure that basic health care services are made available to the masses to achieve the objectives of health for all. In practice therefore, no government (including Nigeria) has enough financial sources needed to meet the health needs of the population. For this reason, a new strategy for health care delivery system is worth considering, for it is a determination of the government to bring health care within the reach of every one particularly the under privileged who have been left out of health (FMOH, 2004).

Benue state today as in most parts of Nigeria is faced with high population growth, high poverty level accompanied by illiteracy and ignorance, poor nutrition, rampant superstitious beliefs, taboos and other related health risk and problems such as inadequate sanitation, unsafe drinking water and high rate of environmental pollution. These conditions have encouraged high prevalence cases of both infant and adult diseases such as measles, diarrhea, tuberculosis, cardio vascular diseases and other respiratory infections. Also, deadly diseases such as Human Immune Deficiency Virus/Acquired Immune Deficiency Syndrome (HIV/AIDS) and other Sexually Transmitted Diseases/Sexually Transmitted Infections. (STDs/STIs) are particularly worrisome in Kaduna State (Laah and Mamman, 2002). There is also growing number of child mortality aged 0-4 years, maternal mortality is also high. Consequently, life expectancy is lower than expected. It is therefore necessary that we understand the vital role of health in both the curative and most especially the preventive services of our health care delivery system. It is against this background that this study on PHC in Benue State is being carried out. The study

4

attempts to explore the impact and challenges of PHC delivery system with the intension of generating data for policy and planning.

The goal of primary health care (PHC) was to provide accessible health for all by the year 2020 and beyond. Unfortunately, this is yet to be achieved in Nigeria and seems to be unrealistic in the next decade. The PHC aims at providing people of the world with the basic health services. Though PHC centers were established in both rural and urban areas in Nigeria with the intention of equity and easy access, regrettably, the rural populations in Nigeria are seriously underserved when compared with their urban counterparts. About two-thirds of Nigerians reside in rural (http.//www.fao.org/countryprofiles/ index.asp) areas therefore they deserve to be served with all the components of PHC. Primary health care, which is supposed to be the bedrock of the country's health care policy, is currently catering for less than 20% of the potential patients (Gupta et al., 2004). While most PHC facilities are in various state of disrepair, with equipment and infrastructure being either absent or obsolete, the referral system is almost non-existent. The goal of the National Health Policy (1987) is to bring about a comprehensive health care system, based on primary health care that is promotive, protective, preventive, restorative and rehabilitative to all citizens within the available resources so that individuals and communities are assured of productivity, social well- being and enjoyment of living. The health services, based on PHC, include among other things: education concerning prevailing health problems and the methods of preventing and controlling them, promotion of food supply   and   proper nutrition, material and child care, including family planning immunization against the major infectious diseases, prevention and control of locally endemic and epidemic diseases and provision of essential drugs and supplies. The provision of health care at PHC level is largely the responsibility of local governments with the support of state ministries of health and within the overall national health policy (Nigeria Constitution, 1999). Private medical practitioners also provide health care at this level. Although PHC was said to have made much progress in the 1980s, its goal of 90% coverage was probably excessively ambitious, especially in view of the economic strains of structural adjustment that permeated the Nigerian economy throughout the late 1980s. But many international donor agencies such as UNICEF, World Health Organization (WHO) and the United States Aids for International Development, (USAID) embraced the programme and participated actively in the design and implementation of programmes at that level (USAID, 1994). At a stage, most of the programmes were donor driven. It was not surprising that at the height of the political crisis in 1993, most of them withdrew their funding and the programme started experiencing hiccups. With the return to democracy in 1999, however, primary health care system deteriorated to an unacceptable level.

The availability of basic health services provided by the PHC especially to rural areas in a country might be used as a yardstick to measure the extent of its health level of development. The aim of this seminar is to describe some strategies which, if implemented, might enhance the proper and timely use of PHC by Nigerian rural populations.

1.2 Statement of Problem

The PHC system currently faces a number of challenges including funding constraints and ineffective management. Although management of PHCs constitutionally falls within the purview of the 3rd tier of government (Local Government Area), poor funding due to the skewed federal allocation system in the country and lack of prioritization of healthcare by the local government administrators has rendered most of the PHCs ineffective. Realizing the importance of Primary Health Care centres to meeting the health needs of rural dwellers and also to help advocate for improved health care services across its project states, LGAs and communities. The essence of health care to the local government is to make the management of PHC services more effective and closer to the grassroots. However, in view of the level of health awareness, one begins to question the extent to which health care has been taken to the doorstep of the rural people. One of the hindrances to the development of health especially in Benue and Nigeria in general has to do with insufficient number of medical personnel as well as their uneven distribution. The Third Development Plan (1975 to 1980) for Nigeria focused on the inequity in the distribution of medical facilities and manpower/personnel. Despite the desire by the government to ensure a more equitable distribution of resources, glaring disparities are still evident. The deterioration in government facilities, low salaries and poor working conditions had resulted in a mass exodus of health professionals (Iyun, 1988). There has been too much concentration of medical personnel at the urban to the neglect of the rural areas. Another significant problem in the management of PHC is transportation. It has been reported in LGA PHCs that there are not enough vehicles for workers to perform their task especially to the rural areas. Immunization outreach services are inadequately conducted. The maintenance culture of the existing vehicles is poor while PHC vehicles were used for other purposes other than health related activities. To put succinctly, many of the PHC vehicles donated by UNICEF in the 1980s are totally non- functional (Wunsch and Olowu, 1996). Access to many parts of the communities is a function of: natural topographical and weather conditions inadequate finance; over dependence of the LGA on federal, state and international agencies for support - the internally generated revenue of the LGA is meager (Adeyemo, 2005); low level of community involvement (Omoleke, 2005), general misuse and abuse of the scarce resources by some political and administrative leadership and high leadership turnover at LGAs (Adeyemo, 2005).

Based on the forgoing,this paper raises the following questions are raised to do justice to the issues.

i.   To identify the level of poor condition in primary health care facilities in Benue state

ii.   To assess the relationship between quality health personnel and primary health care delivery services In Benue state

iii. To assert if there is PHC system currently faces a number of challenges including funding constraints and ineffective management Benue state

1.3   Objectives of the Study

The broad ojective of the study is to examine the Primary health care delivery:Issue and challenges.The specific objective include

i.   To verify the level of poor condition in primary health care facilities in Benue state

ii.   To investigate the relationship between quality health personnel and primary health care delivery services In Benue state

iii. To analyze if there is PHC system currently faces a number of challenges including funding constraints and ineffective management Benue state

1.4   Implications of the study

The study is basically aimed to fulfill an academic requirement as a partial fulfillment for the seminar course unit for the award of a Doctor of philosophy in Public Administration. Nevertheless,it is hoped that it would go a long way to encourage more meaningful document to policy makers and administrators especially as it regards the needs to imbibe goal of primary health care (PHC) as to provide accessible health for all in both private public health institutions.It is also hoped that this paper will be an eye opener to government who over time has thrown the issues of primary health care delivery into trash.It is hoped that imbibing the recommendation of this paper will improve organizations as a whole lot

7

SECTION TWO: REVIEW OF RELATED LITERATURE

2.1 Conceptual Review

2.1.1 The Concept of Health

In the constitution of the World Health Organization, health is defined as a state of complete physical, menial and social well-being, and not merely the absence of disease or infirmity (Jegede, 2010). Physical health is the overall condition ot a living organism at a given time. It involves the soundness of the body, freedom from disease or abnormality, and the condition of optimal well-being. Physical health could be determined *by* several factors. Genetic **malfunctioning** and environmental factors could account for the inability of human body to function as designed. Mental health has long existed as one of the major components

2.1.2 Primary health care

Primary Health Care has been identified as the most basic and probably most important aspect of healthcare because it touches the largest segment of the population-the poor, especially the rural dwellers. Primary Health Care (PHC) is an essential health care based on practical, scientifically sound and socially acceptable methods and technology, made universally accessible to individuals and families in the community through their full participation and at a cost that the community and country can afford to maintain at every stage of their development in the spirit of self-reliance and self-determination"10. The Alma-Ata Declaration of 1978 evolved as a result of the challenges facing health care particularly at the primary health care level which if not addressed will hamper the realization of the goal of „Health for All". It aims at addressing the main health problems in the communities by providing promotional, preventive, curative and rehabilitative services. This triggered the restructuring of the Nigerian health system to align with the Alma Ata declaration-being one of the 134 signatory to the idea. The implementation of primary health care in Nigeria however varies based on the PHC type11. Taking cognizance of the aforementioned facts, the Nigerian government is strongly committed to strengthening the delivery of primary health care services to ensure universal coverage and access. This commitment is articulated in several frameworks such as the National Strategic Health Development Plan (NSHDP), the National Primary Health Care Development Agency Minimum Package of Care, the Integrated Maternal, New-born and Child Health Strategy, the National Health Insurance Policy and the National Health Bill to mention a few12. Implementing these frameworks however, requires a collaborative effort of several ministries, departments and agencies (MDAs), development partners and private sector in an integrated approach to meeting the needs of the Nigerian people, particularly those in (poor) rural areas where the health indices are relatively worse. Currently, the PHC system faces many challenges including funding constraints and ineffective management. PHC constitutionally is a responsibility of the 3rd tier of government (Local Government Area). However,due to the skewed federal allocation system in the country, poor funding of the LGAs in addition to the fact that successive local government administrators have not been prioritizing healthcare, the PHCs have been left unattended to. The identified problems notwithstanding, the provision of quality healthcare is a social responsibility of the Government and any inadequacy at the PHC level will automatically translate to a fracture of secondary and tertiary healthcare, which impacts negatively on both State and Federal tiers of Government. In order to circumvent these, the Federal Government set up the National Primary Health Care Development Agency and consequently the States versions to ameliorate this problem.

2.2 Contextual Review

2.2.1 Critical issues in Primary Health Care Services in Nigeria

The Nigerian government is committed to quality and accessible public health services through provision of primary health care (PHC) in rural areas as well as provision of preventive and curative services (Nigeria Constitution, 1999). PHC is provided by local government authority through health centers and health posts and they are staffed by nurses, midwives, community heath officers, heath technicians, community health extension workers and by physicians (doctors) especially in the southern part of the country. The services provided at these PHCs include: prevention and treatment of com- municable diseases, immunization, maternal and child health services, family planning, public health education, environmental health and the collection of statistical data on health and heath related events. The health care delivery at the LGA is headed politically by a supervisory councilor and technically and administratively by a PHC coordinator and assisted by a deputy coordinator. The PHC co-coordinator reports to the supervisory councilor who in turn reports to the LGA chairman (Adeyemo, 2005; Federal Ministry of Health, 2004). The different components of the LGA PHC are manned by personnel of diverse specialty. The LGA is running her primary health care services delivery in compliance with the principles / framework of the National Health Policy (Nigerian National Health Bill, 1987). The LGA is divided into various health districts/wards so as to enhance maximum benefit of the principle of decentralization of the health sector whereby people are involved, participate and mobilized in the PHC processes.

Problem areas in the implementation of PHC

The essence of health care to the local government is to make the management of PHC services more effective and closer to the grassroots. However, in view of the level of health awareness, one begins to question the extent to which health care has been taken to the doorstep of the rural people. One of the hindrances to the development of health especially in Nigeria has to do with insufficient number of medical personnel as well as their uneven distribution. The Third Development Plan (1975 to 1980) for Nigeria focused on the inequity in the distribution of medical facilities and manpower/personnel. Despite the desire by the government to ensure a more equitable distribution of resources, glaring disparities are still evident. The deterioration in government facilities, low salaries and poor working conditions had resulted in a mass exodus of health professionals (Iyun, 1988). There has been too much concentration of medical personnel at the urban to the neglect of the rural areas. Another significant problem in the management of PHC is transportation. It has been reported in LGA PHCs that there are not enough vehicles for workers to perform their task especially to the rural areas. Immunization outreach services are inadequately conducted. The maintenance culture of the existing vehicles is poor while PHC vehicles were used for other purposes other than health related activities. To put succinctly, many of the PHC vehicles donated by UNICEF in the 1980s are totally non- functional (Wunsch and Olowu, 1996). Access to many parts of the communities is a function of: natural topographical and weather conditions (http:// en.wikipedia.org/wiki/Geography_of_Nigeria); inadequate finance; over dependence of the LGA on federal, state and international agencies for support - the internally generated revenue of the LGA is meager (Adeyemo, 2005); low level of community involvement (Omoleke, 2005), general misuse and abuse of the scarce resources by some political and administrative leadership and high leadership turnover at LGAs (Adeyemo, 2005).

2.2.2   Health needs and problems of rural populations

There are three health care delivery systems in Nigeria (primary, secondary and tertiary).There are innumerable problems within primary health care delivery system which affect the whole population. An assessment of these problems and needs is important to assure easy accessibility to health care services by rural people. Apparently, people living in remote areas show an adaptability that allows them to adjust to the adverse conditions. Critical observation of some groups of nomads, for example the Fulanis and fishermen from the core northern states, the migrant Tiv farmers from Benue State, reveals satisfactory physical health and increasing resistance to disease or illness, but they are not without health problems. The health and health-related problems of nomads, migrant farmers and rural people include the following:

i. Poverty associated with poor housing, unsatisfactory environmental sanitation, polluted water and food which predispose to malnutrition and infectious diseases. ii. Uneven distribution of health services, and shortage of physicians, nurses and trained health personnel in rural areas. iii. High mortality and low average life expectancy, due to lack of access to health services. It is unfortunate that systematically collected data are lacking about levels of morbidity and mortality in rural communities. Despite the availability of PHC services, some rural dwellers in Nigeria tend to underuse the services due to perceptions of poor quality and inadequacy of available services (Sule et al., 2008). Various reasons can be adduced for the underuse of the services provided: a) difficulties associated with transportation and communications; b) high rates of illiteracy among rural peoples ; c) traditional conservatism and resistance to ideas from outside; deep rooted traditions and customs, including health beliefs and practices, which increase the patronage of the services of traditional healers; and d) lack of understanding of PHC among health professionals and decision-makers resulting in poor quality services; and e) heath worker attitude to work (frequent abstinence from the work place) (Adeyemo, 2005). iv. A tendency to press older children into adult responsibilities early, resulting in psychological problems due to role conflicts. v. Endemic diseases prevalence, such as malaria and trachoma. vi. Zoonotic diseases as a result of their close contact with animals as part of their way of life. Clearly most of the problems and needs of rural areas are multifactoral in origin and require multidisciplinary interventions (Abiodun et al., 2010).

2.3 Strategies for Enhancing the use of PHC Services by Rural Communities

Operational strategy

A comprehensive baseline survey using rapid appraisal techniques should be planned in the initial stages to collect information about the health status, socio- demographic variables, civic amenities, existing health facilities as well as the attitudes and beliefs of the target population towards PHC services.

Reviewing and restructuring of PHC services

Public health goals at all levels of government are influenced by demographic and background variables. In view of this, information about community felt needs becomes paramount. These needs should be properly evaluated and coordinated with different sectors and incorporated into existing PHC services. In addition, new programmes should be developed to meet their unfulfilled needs. Some PHC centers are badly located in terms of physical accessibility. Accessibility can be improved by either relocation of the existing PHC centers, or adding more centers at the village level to bring the services within walking distance of the population of the catchment area. It is essential that PHC personnel are trained and re-trained to orientate people towards the concept and principles of PHC. Likewise, the skills of traditional birth attendants and voluntary village health workers should be enhanced by adequate and pertinent training. Mobile health services intended to meet the needs of the remotest population have proved ineffective and rather too costly. In summary, such mobile services are not cost-effective. The establishment of health centers to serve remote populations would be a better strategy. If need be, working hours of the PHC centers should be adjusted and more emphasis be placed on the care of specific groups, such as mothers, children and the elderly. Therefore, PHC services should be based on fixed structures with a reasonably wide coverage, sufficient flexibility and adequate mobile capacity to fulfill their obligations to all sectors in the population, especially the highly migrant population. Legislation should be enacted for special services like immunization and reproductive health. Family health file/card should be prepared with all information related to health, so that they can be taken by families on the move from one place to another for quick acceptance, greater access and prompt management. Village health committee should be restructured and revitalized to include health personnel, community members, including nomadic people, and women.

Periodic evaluation of PHC centers with regards to the impact of new health programmes and policies. Secondary-level health care facilities should be empowered to monitor and supervise

PHC services. The secondary health facilities should also have some disciplinary authority on erring PHC centers.

Community Participation and involvement

It is almost universally acknowledged by national and international health planners that community participation is the key to the successful implementation of primary health care (PHC). The 1978 Declaration of Alma-Ata identified community participation as 'the process by which individuals and families assume responsibility for their own health and welfare and for those of the community, and develop the capacity to contribute to their community's development (World Health Organi- zation, 1978). Nigeria is one of the few countries in the developing world that has systematically decentralized the delivery of basic services in health to locally elected governments and community based organizations. Com- munity participation has been institutionalized through the creation of village development committees and district development committees that are grass-roots organiza- tions expected to work closely with local governments in monitoring and supporting primary health care services. Recently, there have been several governmental initiatives to strengthen these institutions of community participation to improve health services (World Bank, 2003). The National Health Policy in Nigeria emphasizes active community engagement in the provision of PHC services in the spirit of the Bamako Initiative of 1987, when Health Ministers from various African nations adopted resolutions for promoting sustainable primary health care through community participation in financing, maintenance, and monitoring of services. Community participation was institutionalized in Nigeria through the creation of District Development Committee (DDC) and the Village Development Committee (VDC) (World Bank, 2003). There is a large and growing body of evidence (Mike, 2010) that certain types of service delivery are enhanced with the active participation of the communities they serve. As end-users of the services, communities have a stake in ensuring that services are well-provided, and are also well-positioned to monitor the quality of services. With the benefit of local information, they can assess the specific obstacles facing facilities in providing services and they can seek to ensure that facilities have the necessary infrastructure, supplies and staff motivation to provide the services they are supposed to provide. Some of this can be done through volunteer efforts, such as donations for buying supplies, but most of the benefits of community participation can only be harnessed if there are specific mechanisms in place to enable them to do so. For example, whether or not they are allowed to raise local resources will affect their ability to ensure a smooth flow of supplies. Similarly, whether or not they have a say in the evaluation and rewards/sanctioning of facility staff will affect the extent to which they are able to translate their observation of staff behavior into improved staff responsiveness to local needs.In planning the community participation aspects of primary health care, the collaboration of an anthropologist or rural sociologist with field experience is recommended. Promoting community participation is a skill which must be taught to community health workers, and backed up with support services. The genuine commitment of medical staff to community self help is crucial to the motivation process. Motivation within the community quickly breaks down if materials, expertise, and salaries fail to arrive when promised. Community activities are most successfully promoted with reference to the people's own ideas of purity/pollution, cleanliness/dirtiness, and health/illness. Guidelines for successful community participation include: projects undertaken should be ones that the community has identified as a priority; demonstrations and activities to promote health might be linked with agricultural initiatives, adult literacy campaigns, or programs from other sectors; and it is necessary to make sure the community fully understands all the costs in labor, time, money, and materials. If projects or long term community health programs fail, a quick, simple analysis should be made of constraints that may be operating. Apart from providing health care services based on their expertise, community also help in ensuring professional commitment to achieving the goal of health for all. In the last three decades, there has been an increasing demand for a shift of emphasis from acute care to the prevention of disease and promotion of health, education and research. Health workers should try to achieve the maximum possible while trying to solve other deep-rooted problems so as to make health the right of every individual. Professionals working in outreach areas need to develop confidence and expertise in making decisions, even under extreme conditions. It is advisable to accord suitable rewards and recognition for work under difficult and rigorous conditions to boost the morale of the workers. In rural areas, PHC centers are assisted and manned by local people who are selected and trained in addition to the trained medical personnels from outside the locality. In order to strengthen the interest of these people and ensure their retention in the rural areas special incentives should be given, for example, financial inducement of trained nurse aides or midwives to migrate to rural areas and thereby be permanently available to work. Increased awareness of the public, but especially of nomads and rural communities, about health problems, as a result of encouragement and stimulation from health professionals, leads to the mobilization of community resources and greater control over the social, political, economic and environmental factors which affect global health. This is necessary because health begins at home and in the work place. It is where people live and work that health is made or neglected. So the involvement of the community in devising health plans cannot be over-emphasized. The participation of the public in defining problems, planning, implementation and evaluation of community resources makes them feel responsible, not only for their own health, but also that of others. All members of the community can be involved in some aspects of the health programmes. In rural areas espe-cially, the cooperation of local people is fundamental. Their participation can be encouraged by disseminating relevant health information, increased literacy and making the necessary institutional arrangements. Mutual support between the community and the government is highly needed. Planners should realize that individuals need not feel they are obliged to accept solutions unsui-table for them. The approaches to the delivery of PHC for rural populations should, therefore, be practical and feasible. Women from nomadic and rural communities constitute a major health risk group. So, in PHC programmes, if women are actively involved and treated as responsible and concerned members, they can play an enormously effective part, not just in improving the overall health status, but in achieving greater social justice within their own communities as well. PHC, being people-oriented, should make use of all channels through which people express their concerns over health and health supportive policies and programmes. A social climate can be created in which various groups in society accept the health practices recommended, and thereby help individuals make wiser choices. An enlightened community (that is, a public that knows its rights and responsibilities, supported by political will and awareness at all levels of government) holds the key to making health for all a reality.

2.4 Advocacy and political support/ commitment for health equity

A concern for health equity is not new in global health. Equity was central to the World Health Organization (WHO) 1946 constitution, and to the work that culminated in the Declaration of Alma Ata in 1978. Despite this, the health agenda has mostly focused on securing progress on priority challenges. This has contributed to substantial advances in average life expectancy in most parts of the world. Yet the global health community has often seemed unable to counter the widening inequities brought by uneven progress. The World Health Assembly has the potential to be a turning point in addressing health inequities. Two resolu-tions should be passed, and they should fundamentally have concern for equity and social justice – one on „primary health care, including health systems strengthening" and another on „reducing health inequities through action on the social determinants of health. It can seem a long way from a high-level policy review to action that makes a difference on the ground. Three points are important here. First, health inequities are associated with social inequalities.

Health outcomes are linked to position in social hierarchies, described by income, occupation and education, by ethnic group or by gender and to geographic location, for example, rural or urban. In particular, poor health outcomes are likely where social inequalities intersect, for example, for children of women with no education in poor households in rural areas. Studies (Lucas and Gilles, 1984) in low and middle income countries in Africa and Asia show a stepwise increase in under-five mortality across households by wealth, with children from the poorest fifth of households more likely to die before their fifth birthday than the next poorest and so on across the distribution. This pattern is seen for a number of health outcomes and is known as the social gradient in health, meaning that health outcomes are associated with people"s position in the social hierarchy. The social gradient has important implications for policy as it means that policies and programmes must not only target the worst off in society, but must also address the conditions of the whole of society in order to tackle the gradient in health. Second, and crucial to the social determinants of health approach, is that where differential health outcomes are linked to social inequalities, then action to improve health outcomes must include action to reduce social inequalities. Seen in this light, every sector is, in effect, a health sector, because every sector, including finance, business, agriculture, trade, energy, education, employ- ment, and welfare, impacts on health and health equity. Thirdly, health workers at the heart of communities have a pivotal role to play in raising awareness and calling for action on social determinants and in the process of developing and evaluating action at local and national level. A clear political commitment to health for all and to equity in all sectors is essential to tackle the existing inequalities in the provision of health. Health policy makers and planners should note that health and its maintenance is a major social investment. Formal support from the government and community leaders is required to re-orientate national health strategies, especially the transfer of a greater share of resources to underserved populations. Authority should be given to local administrations regarding decisions about matters related to local needs. Those in power need to go to the people in order to receive and hear their complaints and take the necessary steps to solve them, especially in rural and nomadic settlements. Political commitment is a crucial factor in the process of policy formulation and implementation to ensure adequate services to the neglected sections of society (World Health Organization, 1991). Political environment plays a significant role in making accessible to every person the complete range of health, psychological and social services, including prevention and rehabilitation, thus meeting the needs of underserved individuals, families and special groups. Unfortunately/ surprisingly, health planners in Nigeria have not realized this need. Government must first make the PHC centers attractive by putting up clean structures and equipping them with the right tools, personnel as well as drugs. There is need for total turn around of many of the PHCs. In a bid to strengthen the primary health care, the government should also pass the National Health bill. The bill should aim to establish a framework for the regulation, develop- ment and management of the national health system and underpins primary health care as the entry point into the national health system. The bill should also establish a Primary Healthcare Development Fund, which shall see to the provision of basic health care to as many as possible through the National Health Insurance Scheme. The fund should be administered by the National Primary Health Care Development Agency (NPHCDA). The bill should also provide that funding for the Primary Health Care Development Fund should come from "an amount not less than two per cent of the value of the Consolidated Revenue Fund as well as grants from international donor partners." The bill should stipulate a sharing formula in the utilisation of the fund to the effect that "fifty percent of the amount in the fund would be expended on basic health care for all citizens," while 25% of the fund would be used to provide essential drugs for primary healthcare and 15% of the fund should be used in providing and maintaining logistics used under the primary health care system. The remaining 10% of the fund should be utilized in building human capacity used under the primary healthcare system. The bill should also set guidelines for states and local governments to benefit from the fund. The bill should authorize the state to provide at least ten percent of the cost of the project envisaged while local governments should contribute 5% of the cost of the project. As part of efforts to revitalize the PHC sector and to facilitate the establishment of the Ward Health System, the federal government through the National Primary Health Care Development Agency should complete the construction of model health centers in various needy political wards across the country. There should be also be a 5-year developmental plan to construct model health centers in all political wards in the country

Awareness creation

There is a need for a national approach to health education/promotion/behavior change. Currently, the unit within the PHC responsible for health promotion needs to be supported and strengthened to discharge her responsibilities effectively. Community-based activities should support increased family participation in their own health care. This should include educating them on what services they should expect from PHC, as well as activities/messages on promotion of healthy lifestyles and prevention and early treatment of common illnesses. The PHC should address several aspects of communications/health promotion linked to building awareness and achieving behavior change. It should include communications approaches directed at the family and community level. To enhance the utilization of the health services by people, it is most important that they should recognize the need for such services. This need will only be felt if they start to value health as a worthwhile asset (Morley et al., 1983). For this, they need adequate, relevant, scientific information and education about health, disease and hazardous environments (Lucas and Gilles, 1984). Maximum efforts should be made to study the beliefs and practices about health and disease prevailing among different tribes and population groups. Traditional healers serve as the best source of information in this regard. Practices should be categorized into those that are clearly beneficial or clearly harmful. The information provided should be expressed in simple but quantitative form (Morley et al., 1983), starting from simple matters, such as personal hygiene, and gra- dually progressing towards more comprehensive health education, fostering behavioural changes and community action for health. The language for communication should be the same as that of the local people, audiovisual aids used must be produced locally and be appropriate, and finally the educational programme should be carried out by trained and experienced personnel from the locality (World Health Organization, 1991). Health personnel must be aware of the harmful effects of rapid intervention. It is easier to change practices rather than beliefs because the latter are deep rooted, especially among the rural people. The commitment of rural people to religion can be utilized to support the health messages through quotation from the Quran and hadith and Bible. Local beliefs can be interpreted to fit in with the desired health practices (Last, 1984). Traditional media, such as folk songs and drama shows, are very useful in educating illiterate people, especially rural women, who need a rigorous campaign to utilize effectively the maternal and child health services provided at the PHC centers. Health information should be available to the public in the communication media they know and use regularly (World Health Organization, 1991). Adequate knowledge and desirable attitudes about health are necessarily accompanied by appropriate practices.

Collaboration and partnership with other agencies

Collaboration in PHC focuses on how to create conditions for health care providers every where to work together in the most effective and efficient way with the aim of producing the best health outcomes. Collaboration with other related sectors in the improvement of PHC as part of total socioeconomic development is very important. It has been emphasized that no sector involved in socio- economic development, especially the health sector, can function properly in isolation (Hegazy et al., 1992). Many social factors such as education, housing, transport and communications influence health (Last, 1984), and so does economic factors too. Therefore, collaboration with the relevant sectors is especially important for worthwhile mutual benefits. Collaborative efforts focused on economic development and progress leads to better health. Educational institutions play an important role in the health status of the community, especially in the field of prevention. Teachers can help in the early detection of ill health in students. Students are used as messengers of health to the community. Literacy programmes have been shown to have a great impact on equity-oriented develop- ment in rural areas (World Health Organization, 1991). The educational status of the mother plays a pivotal role in the health of the family. As maternal education among rural and nomadic groups is relatively lacking, adult educational programmes would be of great help. The mass media can contribute effectively to the dissemina- tion of health messages to the population at large. The health sector must play a leading role in health supportive public policies. Health activities should be undertaken concurrently with such measures as the improvement of nutrition, particularly that of children and mothers. Coordination of health-related activities should be devoid of duplication (Hegazy et al., 1992). To make intersectoral coordination a reality, concerted efforts should be made to demonstrate how ill health and disease are closely related to illiteracy, poverty, poor sanitation and environmental conditions, etc. (World Health Organization, 1991). PHC lay emphasis on health care that is essential, practical, scientifically sound, coordinated, accessible, appropriately delivered, and affordable. One route to achievement of improved health outcomes within these parameters is the formation of partnerships. Partnerships adopting the philosophy and five principles of primary health care (PHC) focus on health promotion and prevention of illness and disability, maximum community participation, accessibility to health and health services, interdisciplinary and intersectoral collaboration, and use of appropriate technologies such as resources and strategies.

Appropriate technology

Technical appropriateness means that whatever policies and procedures are used in the delivery of health care, they should be acceptable to all concerned. When introducing any new technology, the authorities must be assured that it will not contravene the beliefs and should be used in a rational way to satisfy the essential health needs of rural people, by using methods acceptable to them such as the use of oral rehydration fluid in place of intravenous fluid; and standpipes which are socially acceptable and financially more feasible than house-to-house connections, etc.

Supervision

The word "supervision" literally means "to over-see". It implies that someone higher up the scale is watching to see that someone lower down is performing their job properly. As early as the Egyptian pyramid builders, supervisors oversaw teams of slaves pulling huge building blocks into place. Since then, those in power, including colonialists, exerted their influence over others by appointing supervisors and inspectors. This form of supervision was most often focused on outcomes and was usually not open to dialogue and consultation about the process. It often favoured ridicule and discipline to push individuals and communities to perform their duties. And it has not fulfilled its promise to improve primary health care delivery. The more traditional supervisory visit focused on inspection and fault finding. Health workers often received little guidance or mentoring on how to improve their performance. They were "frequently left undirected, with few or no milestones to help assess their performance, until the next supervisory visit, and motivation was hard to maintain in such an atmosphere" (Guidelines for Implementing Supportive Supervision, 2003). While most primary health care services acknowledge the need for some form of supervision, we maintain that effective (traditional) supervision has been an abject failure in most primary health care settings in developing countries. For instance, inadequacy in the quality of primary health care facilities in Nigeria was felt to be the product of failure in a range of quality measures – structural (lack of equipment and essential drugs), and process (not using the national case management algorithm and lack of a protocol for systematic supervision of health workers). This study recommends that efforts should be put in place to improve the quality and use of primary health care in Nigeria by focusing not only on providing better resources, but also on low-cost, cost-effective measures that address the process of service delivery such as supervision (Ehiri et al., 2005). From a feeling of dissatisfaction with the old model of supervision (that is, traditional supervision) emerged a new paradigm for supportive supervision. The maximizing access and quality initiative (MAQ) described supportive supervision as "a process that promotes quality at all levels of the health system by strengthening relationships within the system, focusing on the identification and resolution of problems, and helping to optimize the allocation of resources-promoting high standards, teamwork, and better two-way communication (World Health Organization, 1991)." By 2001, the move away from traditional supervision had begun. Decisions were made by WHO to re-write the training modules (World Health Organization, 1991). This guideline clearly laid out the new principles of supportive supervision. While we believe these guidelines provide the basis for improving supervision in most of the developing world, there is also scope for yet more innovative approaches to supervision. Independence, autonomy, community participation and empowerment without the cultural or political climate to ensure that supervision can be conducted may not create an environment conducive to improving outcomes. Health workers at the periphery are faced with complex problems over which they may have little control, scarce resources, and few problem-solving skills. No amount of traditional supervision will overcome this situation. However, the new paradigm of supportive supervision might – where supervisors sit along side the health worker and attempt to solve the problems together. Our observation and data collection during the supervisory visits to some PHC centers revealed that they were being operated erratically a situation leading to non use by the communities. Worryingly, those placed in the role of supervisor have often lacked the technical, managerial, or supervisory skills needed to carry such a task out well – making it unlikely that supervision would be truly supportive. Therefore, for the supervision to be supportive, the supervisors need to be regularly trained.

2.5   Empirical Review

Silas (2000) examines assessment of the primary health care services and utilization of existing health care services in Igabi Local Government Area (LGA). The aim of study is to assess the impact of PHC services and utilization in Igabi Local Government Area of Kaduna state. Data from the study was derived from the administration of a structured Questionnaire, Focus group discussion and data from Hospital records. A total of 516 questionnaires representing 0.12 percent of the entire population were administered with the help of some research assistants. A total of 435 questionnaires were used for analysis which was carried out through the use of computer software, SPSS version 9, entry and cleaning. This indicates a sources rate of 84.3 percent. The result represents their interaction with one another and their influences on the impact of PHC delivery system. The finding also reveals that 52.2percent of the respondents have PHC centres in their communities while a significant proportion of the respondents (47.8

21

percent) indicate that they have no PHC centres. A total of 83.3percent of the respondents indicate that they have dispensaries in their communities; 12.4 percent said that they have clinics in their areas, while 0.2percent of the respondents indicate that they have specialist hospitals. A total of 0.5 percent each indicates that they have herbal/traditional homes and general hospitals, a total of 0.2 percent for the "others" respondents mention that they have pharmacies, patent medicine stores and insurance hospitals. A very striking finding shows that malaria fever is the major cause of ill health in the area which represents 44.8 percent of the respondents and this is followed by typhoid fever (17.2) percent. The study also shows that 52.9 percent of the respondents are not living within the 0-4 kilometers WHO recommendation of a health care facility. Decision making among the respondents on treatment during pregnancy and childbirth shown that husbands and mother-in-law play a prominent role (44.5 percent), and 41.1 percent of the respondents indicate that antenatal patients wait for many hours (4-8) before they are attended to by a health care personnel. The correlation coefficient indicates that the observed r (0.673) is greater than the critical value of (0.195) at 433 degrees of freedom (DF) and at 0.05 level of significance. Therefore; the argument that there is no significant relationship between income status and utilization of PHC services is rejected. It therefore shows that there is a strange association between these variables. The inference from this test is that the higher the level of income the more utilization of PHC services. This shows that the rural inhabitants, as a result of their low level of the income do not utilize PHC services effectively as those with higher incomes. The mass media and government information services are the most powerful sources of information about modern health care delivery system.

2.6 Theoretical framework

Elite Theory

Elite theory's origins lie most clearly in the writings of Gaetamo Mosca (1858-1941), Vilfredo Pareto (1848-1923), and Robert Michels (1876-1936). Mosca emphasized the ways in which tiny minorities out organize and outwit large majorities, adding that "political classes" Mosca's term for political elites usually have "a certain material, intellectual, or even moral superiority" over those they govern. Pareto postulated that in a society with truly unrestricted social mobility, elites would consist of the most adept at using the two modes of " political rule, force and persuasion and who usually enjoy important advantages such as inherited wealth and family connections (1915/1935). Pareto sketched alternating types of governing elites, which he likened them to lions and foxes. While Michels rooted elites ("oligarchies") in the need of large organizations for leaders and experts in order to operate efficiently, as these individuals gain control of funds, information flows, promotions and other aspects of organizational functioning power becomes concentrated in their hands (Linz, 2006). Emphasizing the inescapability and also the relative autonomy of elites, the three men characterized aspirations to fully democratic and egalitarian societies as futile.

Elite theory opposes pluralism, a tradition that assumes that all individuals, or at least the multitude of social groups, have equal power and balance each other out in contributing to democratic political outcomes representing the emergent, aggregate will of the society. Elite theory argues either that democracy is a Utopian folly, as democracy is not realizable within capitalism.

Classical elite theory gave a clear understanding on how primary health care is affected in Nigeria by denying people access to primary health care especially women and children who are not from the elite class, who are not economically powerful, who are not well educated therefore, are made to face reproductive burden beginning from early marriage, excessive child bearing, diseases as well as maternal morbidity and mortality. Classical elite theory, also explains that power lies in position of authority in key economic and political institutions. Again the psychological difference sets elites, apart as they have personal resources for instance, intelligence and skills and a vested interest in the government: while the rest are incompetent and do not have the capabilities of governing themselves, the elite are resourceful and will strive to make the government work for their benefit.

SECTION THREE: ISSUES/GAPS AND OUTCOMES

3.1 Emerging issues

Infrastructure and Human Resource capacities

Infrastructure Overall, the facilities assessed were in fair condition with requiring major renovation. Only one-third of the facilities have accommodation facilities for staff which can be an issue for effective 24 hour service delivery. There are challenges with power supply with only connected to the power grid. Others utilize alternate power sources such as solar power and generators which incur additional operational expenses. There is minimal provision for emergency transportation. E.g facilities have provision for emergency transportation such as ambulances, cars and motor bikes.

Human Resources Inadequate human resource is a critical and cross-cutting challenge. Community health workers (CHEWs) and junior health community health workers (JCHEWs) are the most available cadre of staff overall except in one state (Benue). There is a limit to the range of services that this cadre is authorized to provide. There is a shortage of pharmacists/pharmacy technicians – none were available. Environment health officers were also absent in majority of the local government making them the second most unavailable cadre of health workers. Training focus has been in the areas of family planning, ANC, HIV/PMTCT, malaria and child services (immunization and infant feeding). Clear gaps in capacity building are in the areas of healthcare waste management, TB and opportunistic infections management, and non-communicable diseases especially diabetes.

Status of Available Services Across the assessed facilities, the most widely available services were found to include: malaria, child services like nutrition, diarrhoea, upper respiratory tract infections etc.) at and new-born care. However, the least available services include youth friendly and TB services respectively. More often than not, laboratory services are not available on-site. In some instances, when they are not available on-site, facilities find it difficult to access these services off-site. Examples of laboratory services in this category include CD4 count tests and ZN smears – though Mantoux tests are accessible in most facilities off-site. The tests that are predominantly available overall are those that utilize rapid test kits. Outreach services are not common, Furthermore, the level of support provided by special programmes and initiatives like the DRF, MSS, SURE-P, CHIS, etc. are low generally, although some local government appear to have more presence of these programmes than others

3.2 Gaps in PHC Services in Rural Communities

PHC centers are filtering units for those who require specialized services at the higher levels of care. Specialized medical services such as radiotherapy, orthopaedic procedures and surgeries are completely absent. There are many variations in the ways that medical care is given to rural people. The psychosocial health of rural dwellers is a neglected aspect of services provided. Gap remains in the knowledge of rural health workers to respond satisfactorily to identified problems. This gap needs to be addressed because patients" satisfaction with health care is an important health outcome which has implications for capacity utilisation. And, in health systems that emphasizes the cooperation and involvement of the community, both in terms of resources contribution and management, satisfaction with health care assumes an important dimension in terms of its implication for success of public health programmes (Hegazy et al., 1992). Some of the health workers are untrained and the trained ones lack the modern concept of PHC practice. Although, in principle, PHC requires intrasectoral and intersectoral coordinations and community participation, they are often lacking when put into real practice. Most of the services rendered lack community linkage and because of this, most community members are unaware of some available services. In general, nomadic women and children especially in the northern part of the Benue are the most underprivileged and chronically neglected segment in rural areas. Study has shown that rural women especially nomads, when compared with the urban population, significantly underuse maternal and child health services (Abiodun et al., 2010).

3.3 Outcomes

Infrastructure and Human Resource capacities Create a hub and spoke model for service delivery among supported facilities. Based on infrastructure and staff availability, certain facilities should be designated for basic out-patient services while others designated (supported and staffed) to provide 24 hour MCH services. This will ensure compliance to NPHCDA and other clinical standards governing service delivery. To support the hub and spoke model, emergency transportation services must be functional, available to and sufficient for facilities within defined catchment areas. These services must be well structured to include a formal referral network and implementation support. Appropriate task-shifting should be encouraged for health workers in line with the new task-shifting policy guidelines to expand the scope of services the lower level of staff can safely and appropriately deliver. Community volunteers can also be engaged and trained to support service delivery at the facilities as appropriate. These trainings can be in areas such as basic life-saving skills, counseling services, medical records, etc. This will relieve the shortage of staff in the interim. Community structures can provide token stipends and non-monetary incentives for these volunteers. Health care waste management and infection control must be strengthened at this level of care.

Status of Available Services Capacity to conduct basic investigations should be strengthened with the use of rapid test kits where available and appropriate. This should include approved kits with high sensitivity and specificity. Also, new innovative approaches and technologies such as blood grouping test kits and MCH combo test kits which combine multiple tests (hepatitis, syphilis and blood group required for ANC) should be explored. Appropriate national and state-level structures and agencies should be engaged to improve programme coverage. These structures include SURE-P, MSS, NHIS and other initiatives.

Utilization and Service Delivery Commodity logistics need to be strengthened. Appropriate government structures need to be engaged in this regard. Innovative approaches can also be explored in the different LGAs such as community-driven drug revolving funds and structured partnerships with local pharmacies/PPMVs to ensure affordable and regular availability of commodities at the PHC point.

SECTION FOUR: CONCLUSION AND RECOMMMENDATIONS

While the PHC centers are relatively uniformly distributed throughout Nigeria, rural people tend to under-use the basic health services. Although there is no single solution to this problem in Nigeria, some strategies have been outlined which could result in enhancing the use of health services by the rural communities. Capacity building and empowerment of communities through orientation, mobilization and community organization as regards training, information sharing and continuous dialogue, could further enhance the utilization of PHC services by rural populations. Quality of care and service delivery must be assured by those in management positions. In situations of scarce resources, it is particularly important to maintain standards of practice when huge demands are placed on staff, often resulting in less-than-ideal behaviour. It is precisely in such situations that staffs need to know there is support from their superiors, and managers need to know that the scarce health budget is being used to best advantage. Primary health care in Nigeria and especially in rural areas have come a long way and certainly still require more effort so as to achieve the goal of health for all now and beyond

Recommendations for future improvement

Having identified the litany of problems against effective and efficient implementation and achievement of the goals and objectives of primary health care services delivery at the local government, the following recom- mendations are suggested as a way forward:

1. There is the dearth need for the Local government as well as all the other tiers of government to increase their allocation to the health sector. Local governments on the other hand should be more inward-looking and aggressive in the area of internally-generated revenue. This is to reduce the dependence on the federation account in financing health programmes.

2. Priority should be given to improved living condition of the people beyond the present poverty level, so as to enhance better healthy living. To this end, intensive and effective health education of the public must of necessity, be reinforced in other to eliminate such diseases as malaria, typhoid and other infectious diseases.

3. There is the need for maintenance of minimum health standard, improved housing condition, adequate potable water supply, environment sanitation and food supply for the sustenance of good health condition.

4. Poor leadership and political instability have been the basis for unsuccessful implementation of most govern- ment policies and programmes on health care delivery. Therefore, good leadership and political stability is desirable to provide enabling environment for the implementation of the PHC programmes. This will invariably reduce the problem of abandoned projects in the health sector.

5. There is the need to put a stop to unnecessary responsibilities being given to LGA"s by the state governments. It is a common occurrence for federal and state governments to shift part of their responsibilities to LGA, such as purchase of nonfunctioning generator, fridges, iceliners and solar fridges and imposition of sponsored programmes. All these are drains on the lean purse of the local governments with its attendant effects on health services delivery.

6. Adequate supervision, monitoring and evaluation of programmes should be pursued with vigor and required manpower provided. The Nigerian health policy makers should give priority to the training of more rural health workers. This is to prevent the drift of rural health workers from the rural communities to the urban centers.

7. More financial and other incentives should be provided to prevent the high staff turn-over of health workers

REFERENCES

Abiodun AJ (2010). Patients" Satisfaction with Quality Attributes of Primary Health Care Services in Nigeria. J. Health. Manag., 12(1): 39-54.

Adeyemo DO (2005). Local government and health care delivery in Nigeria. J. Hum. Ecol., 18(2): 149-160.

Alma-Ata (1978). Primary health care. Geneva, World Health Organization, 1978. Ehiri JE, Oyo-Ita AE, Anyanwu EC, Meremikwu MM, Ikpeme MB (2005). Quality of child health services in primary health care facilities in south-east Nigeria. Child Care Health Dev., 31(2): 181- 91.

Federal Ministry of Health (1987). National Health policy, Nigerian Natioanl Health Bill. Federal Ministry of Health (2004). Healthcare in Nigeria. Annual Bulletin of the Federal Ministry of Health, Abuja, Nigeria. Guidelines for Implementing Supportive Supervision (2003). A step-by- step guide with tools to support immunization. Seattle: PATH. Gupta MD,

Gauri, V, Khemani S (2004). Decentralised Delivery of Primary Health Services in Nigeria: Survey Evidence from the States of Lagos and Kogi, Washington: The World Bank Hegazy IS, Ferwana MS,

Qureshi NA (1992). Utilization of maternal health services: a comparative study between residents and nomads.

Saudi. Mmed.ical Jj.ournal, 1992, 13(6): 552-4. Iyun F (1988). Inequalities in health care in Ondo State, Nigeria. Health Policy and Plann.,ing; 3(2): 159-163. © 1988

Last JM (1984). Maxcy-Rosenaue public health and preventive medicine, 11th ed., pp. 1647-708. Lucas AD, Gilles HM (1984). A short textbook of preventive medicine for the tropics, 2nd ed., pp. 270-273, 320-323

Mike E (2010). Community Participation in PHC services in Nigeria. Available at www.ngnhc.org/. Morley D, Rohde JE, Williams G (1983). Practising health for all. Oxford, Oxford Medical Publications, pp. 319-26. Nigeria Constitution (1999).; Section 7(1)

C. Omoleke II (2005). PHC services in Nigeria. Constraints to optimal performance. Niger. J. Med., 14(2): 206-12.

Sule SS, Ijadunola KT, Onayade AA, Fatusi AO, Soetan RO, Connell FA (2008). Utilization of primary health care facilities: lessons from a rural community in southwest Nigeria. Niger. J. Med., 17(1): 98-106. USAID Governance Initiative in Nigeria (1994). A Strategic assessment   of PHC and local government-USAID Lagos 1994.

World Bank (2003). Decentralized Delivery of Primary Health Services in Nigeria: Survey Evidence from the States of Lagos and Kogi, African Region Human Development Working Papers Series.

World Health Organization (1991) Health promotion in developing countries. Briefing book to the Sundsvall Conference on Supportive   Environments. Geneva. World Health Organization (1991). PHS capacity-building strategies (1991). Public Health Report Series, Geneva, 106(1): 5-15. Wunsch JS,

Olowu D (1996). Regime transformation from below: Decentralization, local governance, and democratic reform in Nigeria. J. Comp. Int. Dev., 31(4): 66-82.

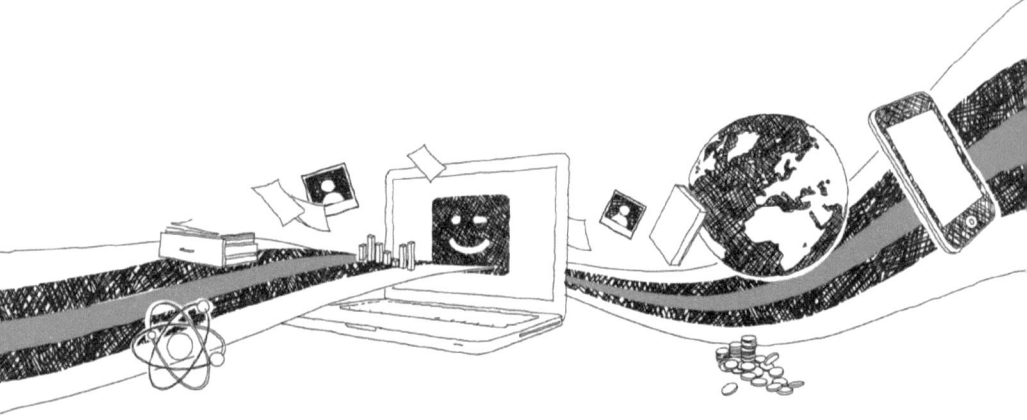
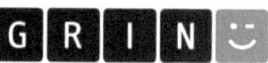